Table of Contents

I0420227

Intro

I want to give you all the ingredients to cook a healthy life, by advocating balance of the mind, body, and soul to reach true wellness. In order for me to help you meet that criteria, I must give you detailed blueprints for each component of the sacred triad. This book will cover the body. Take this as a reminder that humans are living organisms, just like animals. We are equipped with hardware and software (our anatomy, physiology, and genetics), and in order to feel and perform our best, we must optimize them. Physical training, maintaining healthy stress levels, and seeking knowledge are just a few ways we can run our machinery at full force. Even though humans are intelligent and have made technological improvements to make lives less physically dependent, it is important to remember to take care of our bodies so we can better host our powerful brains. As a certified personal trainer with a deep passion to better myself and help my community grow stronger, I want to give you an all-inclusive manual on how to build a badass meat robot. Whether your goal is to lose stubborn fat, pack on muscle mass, get stronger, faster, or increase work capacity, you will be stuffed full of delicious knowledge.

What is "In Shape"?

There are countless ways to view being in shape, but I like to focus on the realms of aesthetics, performance and health. Mainstream fitness is usually portrayed through the lens of aesthetics. Next popular might be performance, with health being the least sexy of the three. Again, integration is of the utmost importance, and being in shape can and should include all three to some degree. A healthy human usually looks good, is strong, and moves well. However, bodybuilders are not always athletic, powerlifters may not be healthy, and health nuts sometimes lose sight of the other two factors. But don't worry, you can be a strong, sexy beast and still eat your veggies.

Instagram fitness pages, and mainstream media are flooded with booties, abs, and yoked dudes. Most of us begin our journey towards fitness based on aesthetics. Everyone wants to look sexy, and popular media supports this premise in the worst ways. Regardless, there is no wrong reason to work out; going to the gym with the goals of losing fat and getting big muscles or a tight booty is a worthwhile mission. The most exemplary figures in this niche are the bodybuilders. In general, these guys and gals are interested in packing on muscle mass, achieving low body fat levels, and sculpting their body around individual muscle development and symmetry. Although usually very strong, their focus is not based on strength alone, but primarily hypertrophy (increasing muscle size). They tend to be very in tune with their nutrition, although sometimes not in the healthiest ways. Some may eat junk food for the sake of shoveling in enough calories to stay 250lbs, and others subscribe to dangerous methods of fat loss, and maintain dangerously low stores. Your goals are personal choices, and I support sexy bodies. So if getting that beach body is what drives you to keep it moving, more power to you.

Performance and athleticism are synonymous in the fitness world. Specific training to get better at football, basketball, etc. and strength sports such as powerlifting, weightlifting, strongman, and gymnastics are all based around engineering the baddest body. Performance never lies, and as Mark Bell says, "strength is never a weakness." If your fitness goals are more general and less focused on body image, performance is probably your best bet. Becoming stronger is going to facilitate muscle growth, better posture, injury prevention, and improved quality of life. Training for performance transfers to daily living more than just packing on muscle in a bodybuilder fashion. Including skills such as sprinting, jumping, climbing, throwing, and carrying are great ways to transform an Average Joe to a well-rounded athlete.
Finally, health is the most noble impetus to step forward and start moving. With the rise of obesity topping 34% of Americans in 2012[1],

---

[1] Ogden CL, Carroll MD, Kit BK, Flegal KM. Prevalence of Childhood and

it's no wonder why people are interested in taking control of their diet and increasing physical activity. A few biological health markers are blood pressure, VO2 max (how much work your heart and lungs can do), cholesterol, fat mass, and physical pain. Getting active in any way and making better food choices can help stop and reverse many health issues. The sedentary lifestyle of modern times is slowly killing off humans.

These goals do not need to be mutually exclusive, In fact they will all play in to each other fairly heavily. Training for perfect balance between the three is undoubtedly going to bring slower progress than a more specific, focused approach. The basis to a successful training program often involves starting with a very general goal and narrowing it down to be more specific over time.

Let's Get Started

In this manual, you will find all you need to begin chasing down your fitness goals. Aesthetics, performance, health; you will find the answers to your biggest questions in this book. I won't promise you will reach your goals, because the effort is on you. But with all the misinformation and scattered knowledge on the internet, your chances of confusion and frustration are high. I was in your shoes when I first started working out, and I had a lot of questions. I read contradictory advice and came away from each article with more questions than answers. Pay attention, tie your shoelaces, and brace yourself for a barrage of knowledge. Becoming an elite athlete takes years of dedication and learning, but so does reaching any fitness goal. This short book will provide you with the knowledge required to achieve your goals and progress you through your first year of training, without the wasted time of scouring the internet looking for answers.

Adult Obesity in the United States, 2011-2012. *JAMA*.2014;311(8):806-814. doi:10.1001/jama.2014.732.

Chapter 1 – Structure

Before you sign up at a local gym, you need to have a fitness goal. Here is a reminder of the three fitness categories: Aesthetics comes down to body composition; you want to add muscle, and lose fat. Performance refers to a specific athletic goal, which is likely some combination of strength, speed, power and agility. Health is achieved by optimizing the body's physiological systems, so that we can improve our quality of life. Quality movement, the ability to achieve most physical tasks, and a well-maintained engine contribute to a fun, pain-free life.

First, let's cover modalities. What kind of exercises are going to be effective, and which tools should you use? Well, since you are a human, natural human movement patterns are going to be the best place to start. This means you'll want to do things that all human organisms should be able to do, like: squatting, deadlifting, pushing, pulling, running, jumping, swimming, throwing, climbing, and carrying. All of these are compound movements, meaning they incorporate multiple joints at once. They use multiple muscle groups and teach your body to move in an integrated fashion. Not only are they the most economic (a deadlift will give you a wide range of training effects versus an isolated tricep extension), but they transfer bet to making daily activities easier. If you sign up at an average gym, you'll most likely be starting off with lifting weights to train these movements. That brings us to our primary means of building a better body.

Bodyweight movements are an important element of fitness. Fall and need to get up? Pushups. Find yourself dangling off a cliff? You're going to need to be able to do a pull up. It isn't completely necessary to get in better shape, but it is very important to master your own bodyweight to a certain extent before moving on to other loaded exercises. Bodyweight training is an effective means of learning proprioception, or the awareness of your body in space and how to move within your environment. While it is true that

6

some of the strongest and even most successful athletes in their field may not be able to do some more advanced bodyweight movements, they are something everyone should be able to do and focus on as a beginner. The basic bodyweight movements include pushups, dips, and pull ups for upper body. Jumps, squat, and lunge variations are fundamental for lower body.

Once you start building strength, bodyweight jazz is going to become too easy. There are three ways to progress once you are easily able to perform dozens of reps with strict form. One, is by variations, wherein you do a modified version of say, a pushup. A diamond pushup has less mechanical advantage and relies on smaller and weaker muscle groups. A variation of a pull up could be a one arm pull up. Gymnasts are known for progressing this way with movements such as the planche or lever, which build insane strength and control over the body. A second way to progress is by increasing repetitions. By doing this, each set lasts longer, stimulating the muscles to either grow or increase endurance. Sets of 50 pushups is going to take a lot of muscular endurance, but sets of 12 pull ups cause growth and definition of the back musculature. The last way to progress bodyweight movements is to add an external load to them. Weighted pull ups are the first thing that come to mind. By attaching plates to a weight belt, the exercise has become more difficult. This is a good way to build strength. If you are unable to do any bodyweight movement, use regressions to build up to them. There is something transcendental about achieving your first strict pull up.

Lifting weights is a great way to improve your physical prowess. Every day, we are faced with tasks that force us to move an external load. An external load is anything that is not your own bodyweight. Climbing stairs would not be an external load, unless you had to carry your new television upstairs. So, it makes sense to train the body to be better at lifting things, because bodyweight exercises only serve the body to an extent. When you are in the gym, you have a lot of options in terms of lifting. You might gravitate to people who seem to have already achieved your goals. A young man might walk over to the dumbbell area and start mimicking the jacked dude doing bicep curls. Or a high school boy trying to make the varsity football team might go over to a power rack and begin squatting, because he heard it will make him run faster. The main difference between these two boys is that one is going for a big, compound lift, while the other is starting off with an isolation exercise to focus on one muscle group.

A compound lift uses multiple joints and muscle groups. An isolation exercise incorporates only one joint to focus on developing its corresponding muscle group. With a bicep curl, only the elbow moves, and the exercise targets the two heads of the biceps. For performance and strength goals, compound lifts are king, and isolation exercises assist them. A compound movement such as a pushup integrates movement at the shoulders and elbows and works the muscles of the chest, shoulders, triceps, and even lats and biceps. Every workout should begin with the most important lift, usually a squat, bench press, overhead press, or deadlift, but this may vary given very specific goals. A bodybuilder who feels he is lacking in is quads may begin a training session with an isolated exercise for that group, and a new military recruit who is tested on pushups and pull ups may begin with one of those exercises. Then, you can move on to specific lifts that will assist your main movement, or help strengthen a particular weakness. Isolation work is typically going to best serve you at the end of a workout after performing more basic movement patterns. Isolation work is great for developing individual muscles that are lagging behind and limiting your other lifts. Bodybuilders find great success in isolation movements because they can stimulate growth in individual muscles. In an aesthetic formatted program, assistance exercises may not even exist. An arm day may be comprised of solely isolated work performed one after the other. But as a general rule, build a strong foundation in your compound lifts before exploring any isolation work.

But what equipment should you use? Well let's tackle this in the same sense as before and address it from a practical stand point. The advantage of bodyweight exercises is the elimination of gym membership fees. Making a one-time purchase of a pull up bar that hangs within a doorframe is all you need. After progressing, a pair of gymnastics rings to do dips can be hung from the pull up bar in the same doorway. Novices often find gym memberships as a barrier to entry and don't have the knowledge pertaining what to actually do if they decide to join a gym. Simply doing a few pushups, pull ups, and bodyweight squats every day can be an effective tool to build adherence and doesn't take a lot of scheduling. Working out consistently is a big time commitment, and the easier you make it on yourself, the easier it becomes to stick to a program. Removing obstacles like driving 15 minutes to the gym, overcoming the fear of embarrassment (however, the large majority of gym folk are extremely nice and welcoming), and paying monthly fees by making a small investment in one piece of gear allows you to train in the comforts of your own home. The simplest way to begin your fitness journey is to do as many pushups, pull ups, and bodyweight squats every time you walk through the door that has your pull up rig. Mounting it in your bedroom will get you in shape faster than hanging it in the back storage room's door.

Free weights best mimic daily activities. Do you find yourself picking heavy things off the ground occasionally? Deadlifting with a barbell is the best way to learn to safely and effectively lift things off the ground. Mounting that new TV on your wall? Standing overhead pressing is going to help. As far as gym equipment, free weights like barbells and dumbbells are king. A barbell allows you to lift the heaviest weight, while dumbbells better train stabilizing muscles. Kettlebells, sandbags, weight sleds, and even odd things like tractor tires are great for developing "functional" strength. Functional is in quotation marks because there is a fad in the fitness community that looks down on exercises that aren't compound lifts or a close representation of a movement in everyday life. A lot of complicated exercises and methods have come from this craze. At the end of the day, any exercise can be functional. As long as it helps you achieve your specific goal, then it is functioning to serve your purpose.

Your gym probably has lots of machines. Don't worry, it's not wrong to use them. Cables, cams, plate loaders and the likes are great tools. Not getting the chest development you want with dumbbell bench pressing? Throw in cable flies at the end of your workout. Machines take isolation to the next level, and may be very useful for the growth of a particular muscle or working through an injury. Just remember, while sitting in a chair and pushing two handles might burn out your shoulders, it's not as realistic as standing on your own two feet and pressing a barbell over your skull. If you're training for general fitness or performance, machines should be used after the primary compound lifts. If you're after a physique, machines may take up a larger portion of your workout, but don't forget to hit the big lifts. Build your base with free weights, and fill in the gaps with any other tool that you find useful and enjoyable.

Lastly, we can categorize the most athletic modalities as truly "functional". Again, the term functional is relative to how the exercise benefits your goals. In this example, we discuss dynamic and plyometric movements. Plyometric training is focused on the concept of rapidly producing maximal force in a short amount of time to help develop speed and power. Typically, plyometrics refer to jumping, but include throwing and sprinting. By sending an electrical impulse to our muscles, telling them to contract at absolute speed and power, plyometric training is similar to strength training in regard to being neurologically demanding. Top level track and field athletes will strength train because it helps them develop their ability to generate more speed and power. We can call this kind of exercise functional because it allows us to express many athletic attributes at once. Additionally, plyometrics can work in the opposite fashion by facilitating strength gains, which is why an Olympic sprinters can have a very strong squat. The neural demands on the muscle are similar in strength and plyometric training.

Running is unique. Unless you enjoy long distance running or want to be a competitive marathon, triathlon, or cross country athlete, or partake in a sport that includes much running, I do not recommend distance running for general physical training. Conventional wisdom has you believing that running is the key to losing fat and boosting heart health. In reality, it is less effective for shedding fat.[2] We can't argue the health benefits of long distance cardio, but we can point to high intensity interval training (HIIT) as a vastly more effective method of weight loss with equal health benefits, compared to steady state cardio.[3] If you want to run, use it to supplement your other modes of physical activity.

By now you may have selected your fitness goal and have an idea of what kind of exercise sounds fun. But before you run to the gym, you need to understand the relationship between load, volume, intensity, tempo, and frequency and how they relate to muscle gain, fat loss, strength, and endurance. The load of your weights is simply how heavy they are. Volume refers to how much total work or repetitions you do. There is an inverse relationship between load and volume, so when you increase one, the other decreases. This makes sense, because if you are lifting very heavy, it will be difficult to perform many repetitions. Likewise, if you are performing high repetitions of a lift, the load will not be heavy compared to your one rep max.

Intensity is often used synonymously with load, but they are not the same. It's no surprise that they have been described to be the same, because lifting heavy is definitely intense. But, performing a set of squats for 10 reps can be brutal if you're pushing yourself with a challenging load. Intensity really means the intent with which you execute the exercise. Whether it be a heavy set of squats, pushups for as many reps as possible, or even a 5k run through the

---

[2] Shugart, Chris. "Predator Conditioning." Testosterone Nation. October 28, 2013. Accessed September 28, 2015. https://www.t-nation.com/training/predator-conditioning.

[3] Ibid

woods, your intent matters. Slack off and you'll have no one to blame for your delayed progress but yourself. Go all out, and you'll understand why people claim "no pain, no gain".

Tempo reflects the speed of your movements. Tempo can be constant throughout an entire exercise or can be different between the "up" and "down" phases. A fast tempo typically carries over to strength/power/speed, and will benefit performance goals. Slower tempos, especially on the "down" or eccentric phase of a lift are used to help gain strength and also stimulate muscle hypertrophy. For absolute strength and power, a typical repetition will be a controlled eccentric (but not deliberately slow), no pause at the bottom, and maximum speed on the way up (but this doesn't mean the weight will necessarily move fast if you're lifting very heavy). For hypertrophy, consider taking a 2 second eccentric (down phase), a 1 second pause at the bottom, and a 2 second concentric (up phase) contraction.

Frequency is how often you train. Frequency reflects how long you need to recover, and how long a particular skill or feature can degrade if neglected. Both of these variables are heavily affected by intensity. Higher intensity causes more damage and fatigue and therefore requires a greater recovery period. If you want to get stronger, neurological adaptations need to occur. These neurological adaptations come along with high percentages of a max effort lift, and are therefore very taxing. If you want to grow bigger arms, more microtrauma and time under tension is needed to stimulate muscle growth. This microtrauma can take 3-7 days to repair, so it speaks to reason to train a muscle group 1-2 times per week for hypertrophy.[4]

So how do these four variables relate to your goals? Let's break it down by hypertrophy, strength, and conditioning goals.

---

[4] Contreas, Bret. "The Hypertrophy Specialist." Testosterone Nation. October 27, 2010. Accessed September 29, 2015. https://www.t-nation.com/training/hypertrophy-specialist.

Hypertrophy is the increased size of a muscle. In order to accomplish this, we need to damage the fibers that comprise the muscle tissue. These fibers are called myofibrils, and when we lift, we actually impart tiny tears in them. This microtrauma is then repaired and the muscle grows larger and stronger than before. More microtrauma (to an extent) leads to more muscle gains, so volume is a big factor for success. Train 4-7 exercises per muscle group within 8-15 reps for 3-5 sets, each week, split between 1-2 workouts.[5] With moderate frequency, we give the muscles time to repair before training them again. Different muscles will recover at different rates, so we can train some more frequently than others. Our load will be moderate, at 65-80% of your one rep max.

Hypertrophy: muscle growth
    Load: 65-80%
    Volume: 8-15 reps, 3-5+ sets = 150-200 total reps per muscle group per week
    Exercises: 4-7
    Frequency: Split the 150-200 total reps per muscle group into 1-2 training sessions per week

Strength is the ability to lift heavy but transfers directly into speed and power. It is achieved by training the nervous system to recruit muscle fibers accordingly. When we lift heavy, the nervous system must send a very strong electrical impulse to the working muscles to lift the weight. The faster and more frequently that electrical signal is sent, the stronger the muscle contracts.[6] In order to give the nervous system and therefore the muscle the correct stimulus, we must lift heavy. Our volume will be within the 1-5 rep range, placing our load at about 80-95% of our one rep maximum. Because the load is high, the volume will be lower. We are doing low reps, so it will benefit us to do a higher number of sets. If a hypertrophy

[5] Tumminello, Nick. "A Simple Program for Complex Results." Testosterone Nation. December 10, 2010. Accessed October 3, 2015.
    [6] Dumitru, Luminiṭa, Alina Iliescu, Cristian Dumitru, Ruxandra Badea, Simona Săvulescu, Horaṭiu Dinu, and Mihai Berteanu. 2014. "Physiological considerations on Neuromuscular Electrical Stimulation (NMES) in muscular strength training." Palestrica Of The Third Millennium Civilization & Sport 15, no. 2: 134-139. Academic Search Complete, EBSCOhost (accessed September 29, 2015).

template is 3 sets of 10, a strength program might be 6 sets of 3 or 5 sets of 5. Because the nature of lifting heavy means literally to teach the nervous system to recruit a muscle, training the pattern often will help us lift more efficiently and thus make us stronger. But due to the load and naturally the intensity being so high, training too frequently can halt progress. Some programs call for max effort squats every single day, others only once or twice. Depending on training experience, seasoned athletes can endure higher frequency at maximum intensity. Because strength training is largely neurological, multiple strength sessions per week of a single movement serves as added practice spent perfecting technique.

Strength: ability to lift heavy, be fast, and powerful
       Load: 80-95%
       Volume: 1-5 reps, 3-7 sets
       Exercises: 1-3 + accessories
       Frequency: 1-5 times per week

Conditioning (read as cardio) increases the heart's VO2max, or how much blood and oxygen it can move throughout the body. It is preferably trained via high intensity intervals (HIIT). This means we move as fast and hard as possible for short periods of time, preferably with full body movements. Also called burst training, the focus is to get the heart rate extremely high (75-95% max heart rate). Since there is a high demand on the body during these intense bouts, we won't be able to work for long periods. Try doing an all-out 50 meter sprint for more than 10 sets with 30 seconds of rest in between bouts. You will soon realize that maintaining this level of intensity isn't going to last long. What's great about this style of conditioning is that you can implement many different exercises to achieve a strong cardiovascular stimulus, which better translates to various athletic movements. For example, intervals of squats carry over to increasing specific work capacity for that exercise while maintaining or building muscle. This modality has interchangeable variables with which to play. The load, volume, and even exercise selection is up to your discretion. The goal is simply to work as hard as possible and get your heart rate through the ceiling. Frequency of this training depends on your fat loss, health, or work capacity goals. Trying to shed lots of fat; do this 2-3 times a week. Just trying to maintain a good blood pump? 1-2 times a week is a solid prescription. With high intensity intervals, you will improve specific work capacity, train endurance in various energy systems, improve cardiovascular function, and likely increase power, speed, and muscle mass. Exclusively relying on running indeed burns fat and increase aerobic capacity, but is horribly inefficient at preserving muscle mass. Because muscles are not going through full range of motion contractions against resistance, the body does not have any reason to preserve muscle mass when it is short on energy (ie. in a caloric deficit). It will therefore have an affinity to use amino acids (from muscle protein) to create energy, along with burning fat. Interval training does it all, and requires the least amount of time.

Conditioning: increase work capacity, cardiovascular function, metabolism, and fat loss

    Load: variable; must allow consistent movement through the interval

    Volume: as much as you can perform at 100% intensity

    Exercises: variable

    Frequency: 1-3 times per week

    Tabata: 20 seconds of effort, 10 seconds of recovery for a total of 4 minutes

    EMOM: complete an amount of work Every Minute On the Minute for X amount of minutes (10 burpees might take 35 seconds to complete; rest the remaining 25 seconds and repeat.)

To wrap up our discussion on structuring and formulating a workout, it is important to cover balance. Not in the sense of walking a tight rope (although slacklining is super fun), but using all of the body's muscles equally. A muscle's only job is to contract at both ends and become shorter, thus pulling on its two attachment sites and causing a joint action. Based on the location of the muscle, its contraction will cause either flexion (closing of a joint) or extension (opening of a joint). If we perform the same types of movement patterns repeatedly, we can become victims to pattern overload and muscular imbalances. Take a bench press for instance. If you constantly contract the chest muscles, they are going to become tighter and tighter and actually pull your body into a hunched over, rounded out posture. Add incessant bicep curls to the mixing pot, and we've got a recipe for kyphosis and restricted overhead mobility. To save yourself from developing poor posture and chronically tight muscles throughout your body, be sure to work all your muscles equally with a balance between pushing and pulling in all planes.

A quick note: The body is a kinetic chain. This means that all of the bones and muscles in the body affect one another. If we start at the ankle and one foot is turned outward and the arch caves in, then our alignment between both knees and hips is going to be asymmetrical. When the hips are in different positions, the pelvis becomes unaligned. Subsequently, the spine is no longer in a perfect, neutral position, the rib cage and shoulder girdle get thrown off, the neck compensates by slightly bending, and now you have a headache. The more we stay in balance between all of our anatomical structures, the better we feel and perform.

The best way to prevent overtraining a specific muscle group or movement pattern is to use our entire body and perform all kinds of movements. A push is defined by moving a load away from the body. Likewise, a pull brings a load closer to the body. For every push, do a pull. It doesn't have to be right after each other or even in the same workout. Just as long as the total volume matches at the end of the week, you should be in pretty good harmony. For the upper body, make sure to perform horizontal pushes and pulls, matched with vertical pushes and pulls. A horizontal push and pull would be movements like pushups and barbell rows. A vertical push and pull would be anything similar to an overhead press and a pull up. For the legs, we have quad dominant movements like squats, and glute and hamstring (aka posterior chain) exercises such as the deadlift. Squats are more similar to pushing, while deadlifts are a pull. If you already suspect a muscular imbalance, soft tissue and mobility work will likely be needed at specific tight areas, and you may need to spend more time with the weaker, undeveloped counterparts. This might mean doing twice as much pulling to offset an overdeveloped chest.

Chapter 2 – Mobility and Warm Ups

It is important to prepare the body for physical exertion before diving in. Whether you train first thing in the morning, on your lunch break, or later at night after you crush your daily duties, you probably want to warm up after sitting all day. Even if you stand at work, the body must be primed for exercise. The most important factor in warming up is getting the body warm. Especially in the morning, blood flow to skeletal muscle isn't at full force. To avoid injuries, begin every workout with a warm up.

The best place to start is by moving the body. Even if today is leg day, moving through full range of motion of all your joints and body regions gets blood circulating to the places we want. I am a fan of going through every joint and moving through full range of motion to get things loose. By starting from the spine and working outward, I scan my entire body for any stiffness, pain, or general discomfort. If the term "dynamic stretching" sounds familiar, this is exactly what we are doing. By using momentum, we can move through further ranges in motion and pull the muscles beyond their normal resting length. Neck circles, cat and cow yoga positions, arm circles, high knees, Frankenstein walks, and the likes are great options for a total body warm up. Please do not forget to start with the neck and spine before moving outward. By moving through any kinks in the vertebral column, there is less chance of tweaking it later in the warm up or workout. It's not easy to train heavy squats with a pulled neck muscle. After just warming up individual joints, start moving in the basic patterns. Holding and repping out a few deep squats is going to help maintain and learn the correct movement pattern. A deep squat is a great way to assess any tight areas. Similarly, a few hinges at the hip (air deadlifts), bent over rows, or even mock overhead presses are a good way to see how the body is feeling when performing more integrated movements, without the added resistance.

After exploring range of motion and scanning for discomfort, you want to address any problem areas. Maybe you feel great and notice no tight regions, but I still encourage you to take this time for any corrective maintenance work you may need. If you have any postural issues involving thoracic spine, pelvic positioning, or overhead mobility (which you vary likely do, as these are prevalent issues in the general population), work on them with soft tissue work and activation of deemphasized muscles. Whether you are just sore and a little tight from the previous workout, or you are addressing chronic imbalances, you have two options for soft tissue work. You can static stretch or foam roll.

Static stretching has gotten a bad rap in the fitness industry as of late and is marketed as outdated and ineffective. I have to disagree. While I will address foam rolling in a bit, I want to identify the benefits of this classic flexibility method. First of all, you don't need to buy anything or rig up any gizmos or gadgets. Simply get yourself in a position that pulls the muscle you want to target and relax. Nature has a way of supplying us with everything we need, and many times our body is great at healing itself. The trick to static stretching is using the breath to relax into deeper ranges of motion and let the muscle ease out of tension. If you're grimacing and having rapid, short, shallow breaths, don't try so hard. Ease off a bit until you can take long, slow, controlled inhalations and exhalations. The point to releasing muscular tension is to down regulate the nervous system. Remember the concept of neuromuscular training and how electrical stimulus makes muscles contract? That is the sympathetic system in which the body gets excited for fight or flight. Stretching helps turn that down a bit and allow the body to enter a more parasympathetic state of relaxation.[7] If you aren't breathing deeply, you won't become relaxed, and your hamstrings will never loosen up. Even though foam rolling is proven to be very effective, I have been able to achieve elite levels of flexibility by the means of static stretching nearly exclusively.

---

[7] "Stress Effects on The Body." Apa.org. Accessed September 29, 2015. http://www.apa.org/helpcenter/stress-body.aspx.

The only time I personally bust out the foam roller is when I'm feeling unusually tight or just feel like switching it up. Foam rolling is the lay term for "self-myofascial release". For all intents and purposes, it's a self-massage. Not all the mechanisms have been identified scientifically, but some of the benefits are increased blood flow, lymphatic fluid flow, reduced muscular adhesions (knots), and reduced muscle pain, along with improving mobility.[8] It is an excellent method of downregulating the sympathetic nervous system and putting the body in a more parasympathetic relaxation state on the muscular level. Think about getting a massage when you have a knot in your back. After you've rubbed out that bump near your shoulder blade you feel great relief and have increased mobility. This is no different. With a foam roller or a lacrosse ball, you can pinpoint restrictions and ease them into relaxation when static stretching isn't getting the job done. If you suspect injuries such as a tear or pull, avoid static stretching and focus on self-myofascial release. Static stretching will likely exacerbate the issues, while massage can smooth out any kinks and bring blood flow into the injury.[9] Because both static stretching and foam rolling downregulate the neural drive to muscles, don't go overboard before training. When we lift weights, especially heavy ones, we want to have as much neural drive as possible. Putting our muscles into a relaxed state makes us weaker. For the best warm up, start with dynamic mobilization of all the joints and ranges of motion, and follow through on the specific tight areas with static stretching or myofascial release. Save the majority of stretching and foam rolling for after your training session, when you need to calm your body down and decrease tension and overall stress the most.

---

[8] Cressey, Eric, and Mike Robertson. "Feel Better for 10 Bucks." Testosterone Nation. July 12, 2004. Accessed September 29, 2015. https://www.t-nation.com/training/feel-better-for-10-bucks.

[9] Gentilcore, Tony. "Soft Tissue Work for Tough Guys." Testosterone Nation. September 19, 2006. Accessed September 29, 2015. https://www.t-nation.com/training/soft-tissue-work-for-tough-guys.

The key to making any change on range of motion and muscle tightness is consistency. Whether or not foam rolling is superior to static stretching, I rarely have any muscle tightness beyond general muscle soreness that one can expect from a hard training session. To boot, I display excellent ranges of motion, erect posture, and minimal asymmetries. I believe that my daily mobility practice which is largely comprised of static stretching and deep breathing is the sole contributor to my nimble body. There's nothing special about any of these techniques, besides consistent implementation.

Warm ups do not have to strictly be about getting loose and mobilized. Sometimes, specific muscles or muscles groups are not "turned on" properly for the movements we are about to do, and thus our performance is limited. For instance, a problem when squatting may be that the knees come in on the up phase. This is an indication that the glutes and other hip extensors and abductors are not firing hard enough. If this is the case, doing a few sets of non-demanding activation drills help turn on the under stimulated muscles. By doing banded lateral walks, hip thrusts, or side-lying clams, the glutes are now primed for squatting, without being fatigued. When you go to squat, the glutes will be more likely to fire properly, and now the knees do not cave inward.

Another example is doing rotator cuff warm ups for the shoulder. Band pull aparts in different planes can activate the small stabilizer muscles around the shoulder joint, so you are less likely to injure yourself and more likely to be a beast in the gym.

Finally, do not neglect work up sets. If the workout calls for squatting 5x5 at 225 lbs, your first set should never be 225 lbs for 5 reps. Start with an empty bar, and do a few reps. Add a plate to each side, continue warming up with sets of 1-10 reps. Repeat in moderate increments while reducing reps until you've worked up to your main working weight. By taking the time to hit lower weights, you can focus on technique and get your body further acclimated to train hard. Take these sets just as seriously as your working sets, and be just as explosive and intent on form with the empty bar as you would with a PR attempt. Every rep counts, and forming good habits paves the way towards perfection.

Chapter 3 - Movements

Let's touch on the basic movements again. For the upper extremities, the body can push and pull vertically and horizontally. In reference to a standing position (anatomical position), a horizontal movement is where your arms are at 90° to the torso, or parallel to the ground. From here, you can push or pull. Likewise, a vertical push or pull is when your arms are usually overhead, or down at your sides – your arms are perpendicular to the ground. In this chapter you will learn a host of exercises that cover different paths of motion and serve various purposes.

Fundamental Movement Patterns
Upper Body

Push: Horizontal
Major Muscle Groups: chest, shoulders, triceps
Main Movements:

Pushup

The most basic of all horizontal pushing patterns is the pushup. Because learning how to move your own body is so critical, the first example for all of the movement patterns will be a bodyweight exercise. Pushups teach integrative movement because many different muscle groups must work together in harmony. Not only is this good for strong triceps, shoulders, and chest, but the stabilization needed to prevent the butt from sagging and lower back from extending teaches the core musculature to properly brace for a neutral spine. Strong glutes, lats, and scapula retraction and protraction are just a few other key factors that make the pushup an integral exercise. Not only is this important for beginners, but a solid tool to keep around even with advanced athletes.

A key when learning the pushup is to progress from inclined pushups where you have your hands on a countertop, bench, or other elevated surface, instead of dropping down to your knees to make them easier. While the knee pushup does help people get strong, the inclined pushup is more specific and easier to progress. Pick a height that allows you to do at least 5 reps. Train at this level until you can do 3-5 sets of 10. Then move down to a lower level and repeat until you get to the ground. When doing a pushup or any other horizontal press, don't let your elbows flare out to the sides. Keep the angle of your upper arm at about 45° or narrower (the more narrow, the more difficult), but no wider. It will activate your chest more if you go closer to 90°, but after time, you are likely to incur shoulder damage. Also, a smaller angle will actually be a stronger position in the long run and is the same technique that world record bench pressers in powerlifting implement. Furthermore, lower yourself all the way to the ground so that the bottom of your chest touches the floor first. If you have your hands at about 1.5x the width of your shoulders and touch the bottom of your chest to the ground, your elbows should naturally assume the ideal 45°, angle and your forearms will be perpendicular to the ground. Keep your spine in a straight line from neck to tail by bracing your core, contract your glutes to stabilize your hips from sagging, and you can even squeeze your quads to make a stronger base. Think of keeping your body in an absolute straight line, while the only pieces that are moving in the kinetic chain are at your shoulders and elbows.

Bench Press

If you've gotten well along your path with the pushups, the bench press is the next best exercise. This is where you can develop the most strength in horizontal pushing, not to mention develop your triceps, shoulders, and chest to much higher levels. The basic tenets of pushups apply and carry very well over to the flat barbell bench press. Elbows are still in the same relationship to the torso, you touch at the lower chest, keep forearms in a straight up and down line underneath the bar, and wrists are neutral. However, the shoulder blades are going to stay retracted and pinned between your back and the bench and never move. If you take a power lifting approach, this is the one place where an arched spine is acceptable. By rounding the back, the range of motion becomes smaller when you go to lower the bar to your chest. This translates to being able to press more weight, because it has a shorter distance to travel. To an extent, this is a full body exercise. You want to drive your feet into the ground to create a very stable base, and therefore generate more power. Because you can add increments of weight to either side of a barbell, you are now working with an external load that you can manipulate and use to track progress.

The incline and decline barbell bench press are variations that hit your pushing muscles in a slightly different way. Incline press requires more shoulder activation, while a decline press can develop the lower chest. Guillotine and wider grip variations that flare the elbows are primarily bodybuilding styles that target chest development. Athletes commonly fare fine with this because they use lighter weight and higher repetitions, which makes it less dangerous. However, please exercise caution when experimenting with a less than optimal shoulder position.

Dumbbell Bench Press

There's no doubt that the barbell bench press will get you strong, and this is partially contributed by the fact that both arms are working in unison and your body has to focus less on stabilizing the load. Dumbbell benching takes away that advantage and makes you learn how to control the weight between left and right arms, as each appendage works independently. While it's important to keep the scapulae retracted, there is usually less of an arched spine, if at all. Typically, a dumbbell bench will be used as an accessory in a strength program, and is performed for higher repetitions with lighter weight. But there is nothing wrong at all with having this be a main pressing movement in a hypertrophy program. Some people with shoulder injuries or discomfort find that dumbbells allow their shoulder to move in a more natural path that doesn't cause any pain. It can also be easier to change grip width to narrow benching with dumbbells.

Wide, Neutral, and Narrow Grip

Grip or hand placement width can tremendously alter the way an exercise feels. In pressing, a wider grip will activate the chest more, while a narrow grip will be challenging for the triceps and shoulders. Neutral hand width is obviously a balance of everything and is regarded as approximately 1.5x shoulder width.

Accessory Movements

Accessory exercises don't always have to supplement the aforementioned standard horizontal presses; they can be just as or more important depending on your goals. Classically, these movements are referred to as accessories because they supplement the main movements of a program. In a strength based approach, pushups, dips, or skull crushers will help develop similar motions or muscles that work well towards making your bench press stronger. However, on a hypertrophy program, perhaps bicep curls are a main movement on an arm day, instead of supplementing your rows after a deadlift workout. In general, an accessory exercise is anything that helps you improve your main lift. They can be compound or isolation exercises, too. For horizontal pressing, accessories may include, but are not limited to, dips, dumbbell pressing, pushups (if they aren't already your main movement), tricep push downs, skull crushers, French curls, kickbacks, incline press, decline press, dumbbell or cable flies, or pec deck.

Progressions:

From the most basic level to some more advanced options, the following are a list of progressions for horizontal pushing.

- Incline pushups
- Pushups
- Diamond pushups
- Decline pushups (feet elevated, hands on floor)
- Flat bench press
- Flat dumbbell bench press
- Incline/decline bench press
- Close grip bench

Push: Vertical
Major Muscle Groups: shoulders, triceps
Main Movements:

Overhead Press (strict)

Pressing overhead addresses the other end of the pushing spectrum with a vertical motion. The biggest roadblock to performing any overhead exercise correctly is shoulder mobility. Tight pecs, lats, and biceps along with poor lower back stabilization and upper back mobility into extension can limit your overhead range of motion. If you cannot lie down on your back, flat on the floor, and raise your arms straight back over your head without your lower back arching up off the floor or experiencing shoulder pain, then you should spend some time working on your mobility. Elect to use a few regressions for your vertical pushing exercise.

A basic way to overhead press is with the barbell. Load it up on the power rack and stand underneath it and place your hands a little wider than shoulder width apart. Grasp the barbell and step out of the rack with the bar on your shoulders. Keep your elbows forward so your forearms are directly underneath the bar, perpendicular to the ground. Just like the bench press, don't allow your elbows to flare out to the sides. Make your base as strong as possible by locking out your knees with a hard contraction in your quads. Prevent your lower back from hyperextending by squeezing the glutes and bracing the core. Press the bar directly overhead so your biceps line up with your ears and your head is sitting within the "window" created by your two biceps. The barbell should be directly over your skull so that the load is stacked on top of your spine. No bouncing with the legs or driving under the bar like in a jerk.

Incline Press

If you cannot fully flex your shoulder overhead, an incline press variation will be a good substitute. You can choose to do a dumbbell press or try a landmine press. Separating both arms and doing a single hand dumbbell overhead press can help with mobility, core stability, and shoulder stability too. Pick a variation that works well for your current range of motion while addressing your limitations at the shoulder.

Accessories

Again, anything that helps your overhead press is considered an accessory. Try dumbbell overhead pressing, push pressing, jerks, front and lateral raises, or anything that helps develop your pushing muscles.

Progressions

- Bench dips
- Single arm landmine press
- Incline bench press
- Standing single arm dumbbell overhead press
- Dumbbell overhead press
- Barbell overhead press
- Dips (add weight with a belt for increased resistance)

Pull: Horizontal
Major Muscle Groups: traps, lats, biceps
Main Movements:

Barbell Row

Pulling is important for a strong back and good posture. A horizontal row with free weights typically involves you hinging forward at the hips so that you can pull a weight towards you against gravity. The bent over barbell row requires such a position, and the weight actually moves in more of a vertical path in relation to the ground. Set the barbell up in a rack so that it's about at mid-thigh. Grab a bit wider than shoulder width apart (just enough so that your arms can clear the width of your torso when you pull), pick the bar up, and take a few steps back out of the rack. From here, get your feet set at about shoulder width, and *hinge* forward, keeping your spine neutral and long. Think about sticking your ass backwards and only creasing at the hips. Once you get here, pull the weight towards your body so the barbell hits your stomach. Again, elbows are not flaring out, but staying at about a 45° angle or less. However with the row, we need to make sure the shoulder isn't popping forward. To avoid the ball moving forward in the socket of the shoulder joint, think about tucking your chin and squeezing your shoulder blades together, and keep your chest out as if you're proud of something. If you don't retract the scapulae, you're not pulling correctly and therefore not receiving the full benefits of the horizontal pull - plus you are putting yourself at risk for shoulder injury.

Inverted Row

This is a good way to use your bodyweight for a horizontal pulling pattern. If your gym has TRX bands or gymnastics rings, grab on and lean back while walking your feet forward so that you are suspended with your chest facing the ceiling. Simply pull yourself towards your hands while bringing the shoulder blades together. In this position, think about being proud and keep your chest out to avoid the forward drifting shoulder problem. You can start at a more upright position and gradually move your feet forward to lower your angle to the ground, just like the pushup progression.

Wide, Neutral, and Narrow Grip

Different hand positions work the back in different ways. A wider grip on a row can help target the upper back more, while a very close grip can burn out the biceps and get the lats engaged more than the trapezius. Use each variation to address whatever you think is a weak point in your pulling architecture.

Accessories

Dumbbell rows, chest supported rows, T bar rows, low rows, and the likes are all compound movements that are great for horizontal pulling. Some isolation exercises include band pull aparts, reverse flies, and all variations of bicep curls. These hit the upper back, lats, and biceps.

Progressions

- Inverted row
- Chest supported row
- T-bar row
- Dumbbell row
- Kroc row
- Barbell row (pronated or supinated)
- Pendlay Row

Pull: Vertical
Major Muscle Groups: lats, biceps, traps
Main Movements:

Pull Up

The pull up is the primary test for upper body strength and the quintessential vertical pull. The difference between a pull up and a chin up is grip. A pull up is when you grab the bar with a pronated grip (palms facing away from you). A chin up has the opposite grip – supinated with palms facing you. Chin ups are easier and therefore a great place for beginners to start. With either movement, you want to start from a dead hang, meaning your elbows are fully locked out. Without kipping (swinging or kicking), pull yourself all the way up so your chin is above the bar. It is important to think about driving your elbows down and into your opposite pockets (left elbow into right pocket, vice versa) to get proper lat and trap recruitment. Avoid rounding your back to strain your way above the bar. You want to think about leaning back so you can squeeze your back and shoulder blades tight, rather than stretch it out and rely on your arms to do all the work. If you cannot do a pull up, use a band to assist yourself up by attaching one end to the bar, and slip your foot into the other end. The tension will reduce your bodyweight significantly. You can progress by starting at as low as 5 sets of 1 rep and increasing to 5x5. Then move to a lighter band and repeat. However, because the bands help so much at the bottom of the pull up, and not a lot at the top, they might make you develop uneven strength in your range of motion. This is why you should also use negative pull ups. Jump up to the top of the bar and slowly lower yourself down via one long eccentric contraction (still pay attention to keeping your back squeezed tight, and slightly lean back). Muscles are stronger in the eccentric (negative) contraction, compared to the concentric contraction, so training in this fashion can elicit substantial strength gains. Start at maybe a 3x1 or 3x3 rep scheme and work yourself up to 3x8 or 5x5. Another variation is to do a few sets of max holds. A 30 second negative pull up is a close approximation to 1 pull up. Some pull up machines exist that allow you to rest your knees on a platform that is counterbalanced with adjustable weights. The more weight you select, the less your body weighs. This is actually a great way to train pull ups because the weight is constant, unlike bands.

Pull Downs

Lat pull downs on cable machines are a good vertical pull too. By sitting down and selecting the resistance, you can get very similar effects that pull ups offer, if you cannot lift your own bodyweight. This makes them another useful tool for progressing to pull ups. Most gyms have them, and if your pull up rig is a straight bar, you are limited to only a few grip selections. Lat pull down machines usually have many handles you can clip in to change how your back is worked. Again, narrow and supinated grip is easier and targets more biceps, while a wider pronated grip will be more difficult. Try them all.

Accessories

There aren't a whole lot of vertical pull options between pull ups and lat pull downs, but all row variations help develop the same pulling muscles you need to enhance. Inverted rows are also an excellent way to progress to pull ups, as you have to work with your own bodyweight.

Progressions

- Inverted row
- Band pull ups
- Negative pull ups
- Chin ups
- Pull ups
- Lat pull downs
- Weighted pull ups

Lower Body

Leg: Push
Major Muscle Groups: quads, glutes
Main Movements:

Bodyweight Squat

Start off with bodyweight squats to either gain the strength needed for your fitness level, or to make sure you have basic mechanics understood. The standard "feet shoulder width apart, toes forward, chest up, ass out" approach has good intentions, but many faults. Beginning at the feet, choose a stance that is comfortable to your anatomical structure. Some people can do feet forward at shoulder width, others will need to point their toes out more and take a wider stance. All are fine, but you want your knees to be able to track over your toes. Do what feels comfortable and allows you to assume an efficient position. From here, sit down like you're taking a seat on a toilet. The butt points back a bit, but mainly comes down as you bend your knees. Now while it is best to hit parallel (thigh bone parallel to floor) or below, some people do not have the mobility, strength, or anatomy (if your hip boney architecture is the case, you may never be able to go below a certain level without compromising spinal alignment[10]) to do so. However, depth should be a priority. Even though powerlifting might not be your sport, official ruling dictates that a squat above parallel does not count as a repetition. Before you go down, take a big breath into your belly and expand your stomach and brace your core as if someone is going to punch you, to create a more stable spine. As you descend and ascend, keep your spine straight, but not necessarily upright and vertical. People with shorter legs will be more upright, while long legged humans tend to hinge over a bit more. Avoid letting your knees drift inwards by focusing on driving them apart and

---

[10] "Butt Wink Is Not About the Hamstrings - DeanSomerset.com." DeanSomersetcom. July 7, 2014. Accessed September 30, 2015.

squeezing your glutes on the way up. Your balance should be mid-foot so that you are not leaning too far forward on your toes and not backwards on your heels. Think about leading the ascent with your chest, so that your hips don't shoot up and cause a separation between the fluid motion that should occur as ankles, knees, and hips extend together. If you have trouble with strength, begin with sitting down to a chair or box and standing back up.

Barbell Squat – Front, High bar, Low bar

Once you figure out the proper mechanics of a bodyweight squat, the next progression is to add some resistance. Bar placement changes the mechanics, and can even help some people perform better than an air squat. In general, a front loaded squat like a front squat or a goblet squat will force the torso to be the most upright, with more emphasis on the quadriceps of the legs. A high barbell squat places the load on the back, but high up on the trapezius muscles, near the base of the neck. This is the second most upright squat position with a barbell, is more transferrable to athleticism, and is commonly the preferred technique of Olympic weightlifters. The low bar squat still places the bar across the back, except it is positioned lower and rests on top of the rear deltoids. The moment arm of the torso becomes shorter, requires you to tip forward the most, relies more on strong hips, and is often the strongest squat variation. Regardless of your preferred squat style, maintain a vertical bar path. The straighter the path, the more efficient and strong the lift.

Narrow vs. Wide Stance

Just as in every lift, grip and stance matter. A closer stance will hit the quads harder in most cases and can be implemented in front squats or any variation that has the chest more upright. Low bar squats can benefit from a wider stance that recruit more hip power and overall strength. Pick the appropriate stance for your goals.

Accessories

Any motion that works the quads or the glutes with any semblance of a squat, or in isolation, will transfer to a better squat, bigger muscles, and therefore facilitate your goal. Anything from lunges to the knee extension machine are appropriate choices. As a reminder, compound movements are more transferrable to performance based goals, and isolation exercises are superior for individual muscle development.

Progressions

- Bodyweight box squat
- Bodyweight squat
- Lunges
- Goblet squat
- Safety squat bar
- High bar back squat
- Low bar back squat
- Front squat

Leg: Pull
Major Muscle Groups: glutes, hamstrings
Main Movements:

Deadlift

So, if squatting hits the quads more and we can consider that to be the front of your leg, deadlifts target hamstrings and glutes (aka the posterior chain) as you pull weight off the ground by using the muscles on the back of your legs. The main purpose of learning this exercise is to safely train to pick up any heavy object off the ground. This lift is considerably more important than any other exercise due to its high practicality and utility in everyday situations. Not only is it applicable to your life, but the physical demands on the body make it the most full body movement available due to the integration of nearly every muscle group. If you've ever heard the term, "lift with your legs, not your back", that's essentially what you need to do in a deadlift. A deadlift is when you pick a barbell off the floor and bring it to a standing position. It requires using weights on each side of the bar that are either 45lbs, or bumper plates that are the standard 17.5in diameter.

Walk up to the bar with feet shoulder width apart and the barbell sitting directly over mid-foot (think about having the bar over your shoelace knot). This ensures that the load will be close to your center of balance, making the mechanics more efficient. Now, starting in an upright standing position, stick your ass backwards so that you hinge at the hip. The spine stays long and neutral and doesn't change at all. All of your movement comes from the hips. At a certain point you will feel the tension in your hamstrings tighten to a degree where you cannot hinge any further. This is where you will have to begin bending your knees to drop your butt down until your hands can reach the bar. (Your hands will be outside of your legs for the conventional stance.) Now that you're set up, check to make sure your shoulders are directly over the bar and your arms are completely vertical. You don't want to be leaning forward over the bar. The barbell should still be very close, if not touching your shins. Take a deep belly breath, brace, and stand up while maintaining a flat back. Just like the squat, initiate the pull with your torso so that your hips don't shoot up first. Think triple extension between ankles, knees, and hips. As you come close to a full standing position, squeeze your glutes and thrust your hips forward into the bar to lockout and fully extend your hips. Stand tall with hips extended, but don't hyperextend your lower back.

Sumo Deadlift

If you're having trouble keeping a neutral spine and you tend to round your back at any point in the deadlift, sumo stance might be for you. Instead of setting up with a shoulder width stance, and hands outside the legs, stand over the barbell with a very side stance, toes pointed outwards. As you drop down, you will be doing more of a squat than a hip hinge, and your hands will be at shoulder width between your legs. This position allows you to get your hips lower and closer to the weight while maintaining a more vertical torso angle. From here, the same principles apply. Stand up by leading the movement with your chest to prevent your hips from coming up too soon and possibly causing a rounded back. Squeeze your glutes to lockout, and stand tall.

Accessories

Glute and hamstring exercises are going to help make your deadlift better and of course help strengthen or stimulate hypertrophy to those muscle groups. A stiff legged deadlift is exactly what it sounds like – don't bend your knees. This will induce a long stretch in the posterior chain followed by isolation of the hamstrings and glutes to execute the lift. Hamstring curls, pull throughs, glute bridges, glute-hamstring raises, and the likes are good supplementary work. Besides that, isometric holds for lower back strength and stabilization are beneficial to help maintain a neutral spine. This can include hyperextensions with a pause at the top, or focusing on a flat back with your stiff legged deadlifts or goodmornings.

Progressions

- Cable pull throughs
- Sumo kettlebell deadlift
- Kettlebell swings
- Trap bar deadlift
- Sumo deadlift
- Conventional deadlift

Core

Major muscle groups: abdominals, obliques, lower back

The purpose of having a strong core is to stabilize the spine while under load. Although the muscles in our trunk can create motion about the spine, it behooves us to focus on making these muscles strong and better able to keep the spine neutral. This is why anti-flexion, anti-extension, anti-rotation, and anti-lateral flexion exercises are better ways to train the core. If you're concerned about getting abs, realize that you already have them. Having visible abs is a matter of being lean. Time spent doing situps and crunches are a considerable waste of time and don't help your cause when trying to maintain a neutral spine in a deadlift or squat. However, ab wheel roll outs are brutally challenging for the core. The core is best used to prevent motion in the spine, so train it accordingly. Instead of holding a weight in one hand and bending sideways over and over to get "side abs", perform a suitcase carry wherein you hold a heavy weight in one hand and walk 50 meters while keeping a tall posture and fighting against the weight trying to pull you sideways.

Progressions:

- Dead bug
- Bird dog
- Plank
- Side plank
- Suit case carry
- Ab wheel roll outs
- Hanging knees to chest
- Hanging toes to bar

All of the above covers the basic human movement patterns. You can train them within the parameters of strength, hypertrophy, or endurance by changing the reps, sets, tempo, rest time, and frequency accordingly. The main movements mentioned are all compound and serve to develop a strong movement foundation, but are by no means the most important exercise for every single goal or person. They are certainly the most effective tool for total athleticism, and are strongly encouraged for you to spend time mastering, but know that you have plenty of other options. Again, if you don't have strictly performance based goals, then maybe you will never bench because you get a better chest pump from cable flies. That's fine. The recommended movements are just suggestions because they are the staple human movements.

Plyometrics

Plyometric training refers to producing as much speed and force as possible in a short amount of time. Movements like jumping, sprinting, or throwing are considered plyometric. Because you move at full pace, these exercises are great for developing more power as an athlete. Most of these exercises only require a concentric contraction, where most lifts require an eccentric portion. With a throw, all your energy goes into concentrically contracting the appropriate muscles to launch the projectile. There is no portion where you need to slow down the object, such as in lowering in a squat each rep. This allows you to generate as much force as possible as you accelerate through the motion. The high demands on the central nervous system make this training very similar to strength training. All out 50 yard sprints can improve squatting strength, and increasing your 1 rep max in squatting can translate to a faster 50 yard sprint time. Track and field sprinters, jumpers, and throwers are some of the strongest and most powerful athletes.

So where do plyometrics fit into your workout regimen? If you are a track or field athlete and you compete in explosive events, maybe you spend time throwing or jumping during your actual skill practice (which would likely be separate from a strength workout). For the general public, plyometrics work well for priming the nervous system at the beginning of a workout or on a separate day for conditioning.

Again, producing high speed and power is very much a nervous system task. This is why something like vertical jumps before a squat session can be beneficial. A high effort jump forces the nervous system to rev up. 5 sets of 1-3 is a good prescription for these, with about 1-2 minutes in between sets to allow a full recovery. You want to recover completely between these sets so that you can continue to generate as much power possible each repetition. Now when you begin squatting, your motor units are firing faster and harder, making your squats stronger. The same protocol can be applied to throws to warm up for upper body lifts.

As for conditioning, plyometrics are useful for HIIT sessions. Throwing a ball (that doesn't bounce) into the ground as hard as possible for as many reps as possible in a tabata format is a very intense workout.

Isolation

Isolation exercises were mentioned in the accessories portions of our fundamental movements. As a reminder, isolation exercises are ones that focus on the movement of one joint system and the muscles that cause that specific joint action. Typically, bicep curls, leg curls, tricep extensions and the likes are performed for higher reps rather than within strength parameters. This kind of movement is particularly beneficial for developing individual muscles or even rehabilitating certain joints. They are also a superior way of training for pure size and aesthetics. As far as transferring to performance, spending time isolating components of bigger movements and their constituent muscle groups can have many positive outcomes. Remember, a larger muscle has larger fibers and therefore a higher potential for strength.

Chest

The pectorals are mainly responsible for horizontal shoulder flexion. Think about a hugging motion. Any exercise that causes resistance in horizontal shoulder flexion will isolate the chest.

- Dumbbell flies
- Cable flies
- Pec deck

Triceps

Triceps are the prime move for elbow extension. Straightening out the elbow against any resistance will train the triceps. Different angles hit the three heads of the triceps differently.

- Kick backs
- French curls
- Cable pull downs
- Skull crushers

Shoulders

There are three shoulder muscles; the anterior (front), lateral (side), and posterior (rear) deltoids. The anterior deltoids mainly control shoulder flexion – think about raising your arms out in front of you like a zombie and following through until your hands are overhead. The lateral deltoids allow you to raise your arms up to the side in a T shape. And the rear deltoids move your arms in the opposite direction of shoulder flexion into shoulder extension and hyperextension. The rear deltoids also cause external rotation of the shoulders. You can train all three of these in isolation by moving through their respected joint actions.

- Front raise
- Lateral raise
- Reverse dumbbell/band flies

Back

The back is a very large group of muscles with various joint actions. The upper back consists mainly of the four trapezius muscles that help bring the shoulder blades together. You can focus on them by doing any exercise that causes horizontal shoulder extension. The lower back is built by the spinal erectors. Contracting them moves the spine into extension, creating an arch. You could train them with concentric contractions, but like abdominals, isometric holds will get them stronger for maintaining spinal rigidity. The lats can be targeted in isolation with shoulder extension exercises when the hands are in a starting position of at least 90° of anterior flexion and pulled down with straight arms at the side (0° flexion).

- Reverse flies (traps)
- Shrugs (traps)
- Straight arm pull downs (lats)
- Supermans (lower back)

Biceps

Responsible for elbow flexion, the biceps move in opposition to the triceps and close the elbow joint.

- Dumbbell curls
- Barbell curls
- Preacher curls
- Hammer curls

Quads

The quadriceps group is located on the front of the thighs and correlates with knee extension, very similar to the triceps at the elbow. In most cases, machines will be the easiest way to train the quadriceps in isolation.

- Knee extension machine

Hamstrings

Literally called the biceps of the thigh (biceps femoris), the hamstrings act to flex the knee. However, they also contribute substantially to hip extension in synergy with the glutes. Machines are also the primary method to train them as far as knee flexion, but there are bodyweight and free weight variations available for hamstring development.

- Hamstring curl machine
- Stiff leg deadlift
- Good mornings
- GHD
- Hyperextensions

Glutes

The primary hip extensor, this big muscle group is responsible for any hip thrusting related motion. From literal hip thrusts to deadlifts, hip extension and strong glutes are essential to high performance and aesthetics. Powerlifters rely on them tremendously, but bodybuilders have mixed feelings. Male bodybuilders tend to spend time developing them, but limit their size to appeal to the classic aesthetic build from the Golden Era where large arms, legs, chest, and back come to a tapered juncture at the waist. This means they have "small" yet shredded abdominals and a small set of glutes. Women however typically chase a fuller, sculpted butt. Thus, females tend to spend more time isolating this area.

- Hip thrusters
- Glute-ham raise machine
- Stiff leg deadlift
- Goodmornings
- Hyperextensions

Calves

These guys like to stay little and can be a pain for bodybuilders to grow. Their primary action is ankle plantar flexion, aka standing on your tippy toes. They get a lot of action from daily walking, so you may have to hit them with copious repetitions to get a strong growth stimulus. Regardless of your potentially stubborn calves, pointing your toes down targets them in isolation.

- Calf raises
- Single leg calf raises
- Calf press

Functional

All of the fundamental movements at the beginning of this chapter are functional. We must realize that any exercise that helps us achieve our goal is automatically functional in its own right. Typically, the term functional refers to exercises that have real world application, which is why the fundamental, human-movement patterns are the "most functional". Some more exercises that have daily utility include loaded carries, pulling or pushing a sled, flipping tires, or even more basic things like swimming, crawling, or climbing. Within your program, these can be implemented well in conditioning workouts (pull a heavy sled 50 meters EMOM) or even in a strength session (push a heavy sled 50 meters for 5 sets after squatting). The choice is up to you – there are no rules as to how you decide to implement different strategies, only guidelines and suggestions.

Olympic Weightlifting

The term "Olympic weightlifting" is redundant. Before lifting weights was popular, the sport of weightlifting had been around since about 1900, and it consists of the snatch and clean and jerk. With the advent of modern fitness making lifting weights popular, weightlifting has become a general term for picking up weights and putting them back down repeatedly. To differentiate weightlifting from general fitness, "Olympic" now prefaces the sport's name due to its inclusion in the Olympic Games.

This style of lifting has been popularized by CrossFit as a means to total body enhancement. The basic components of weightlifting is picking a barbell (which was originally invented for this sport) from the ground and putting it above your head. The snatch does this all in one fluid motion which is vaguely similar to a throw that begins with a deadlift. Versus the clean and jerk which separates the task into two movements that combines a deadlift into front squat (clean) followed by essentially an overhead press (jerk).

Although powerlifting, bodybuilding, and even bodyweight fitness are sports, weightlifting is special with the fact that it uses its own special exercises. Powerlifting and bodybuilding use the basic movement patterns to develop strength and or size, but weightlifting implements very special movements. The lifts are what make it a sport. They are extremely technical, and if you decide to give them a go, it is imperative you take time to learn the correct techniques to prevent injury. The nature of the snatch and clean and jerk is raw power. If you have seen these lifts performed (go look up a video if you haven't), you might wonder how someone can put 400lbs over their head, especially when noticing that many of these athletes are not very big compared to other high level strength athletes. It's all in the technique, and much of it has less to do with getting the weight overhead, but getting underneath the weight. This requires ferocious speed, and of course incredible strength.

Naturally, Olympic lifts are a great tool to implement into any strength, speed, or power based program. Again, because they are so demanding, place them at the beginning of your training sessions.

Gymnastics

Gymnastics is the sport of bodyweight exercise. Many, if not all, of the movements are specialized for the sport and require elite body awareness and relative strength (strength to bodyweight ratio). A gymnast might not be able to bench press her bodyweight, but a woman who can bench 135lbs most likely cannot hold a full planche. Whether the event is rings, parallel bars, or floor, gymnasts are some of the best athletes around. This sport is also very strength based, as it doesn't pay to carry excess muscle mass or be able to run a marathon while attempting an iron cross or triple backflip. Gymnasts require top level mobility. The guy that swings around on rings has absolutely no restrictions in his shoulder range of motion. Likewise the girl doing splits on the balance beam can bend into all kinds of twists and turns.

This is yet another available option at your expense to get into better shape and upgrade your meat robot. Structuring fitness based solely on either gymnastics or Olympic weightlifting probably requires going to a specialized facility or hiring a coach, which makes this entire fitness manual nearly worthless to you. However, including these more technical exercises into your training regimen can be worthwhile. Moving in different ways will help keep you inspired, motivated, humble, and hungry for progression.

Chapter 4 – Play

Playing is an integral portion of physical fitness. Working out can certainly be fun and a source of enjoyment, but part of training to have an optimally functioning body is to use it in different ways. The human body is designed to conquer a multitude of tasks, and the gym can only offer so many movement possibilities. If you want to test what your meat robot can do, expose it to unlimited physical puzzles. The gym is very structured and a laboratory in many ways, because you can control every single variable. Life is different and unpredictable, as are many sports.

Getting outside of the gym and playing might not be an issue for some people. A serious lacrosse athlete spends most of his time playing, and in fact probably struggles to fit going to the gym into his busy practice schedule. Some athlete's sport is literally lifting weights, such as powerlifters and weightlifters. In the latter example, playing doesn't occur unless it is built into the athlete's free time. The goal of playing is to move your body in new, mostly random ways.

Playtime is not only about using your improved physicality for solving new, different tasks. It's supposed to be fun. When you find something that is truly playful, you might consider skipping a gym session to do it more often. Oftentimes this activity becomes a passion that drives your training in the gym to focus on getting better for this activity. Perhaps once a week you go on a hike or hit the mats at your local Brazilian Jiu-Jitsu school. Maybe it's not one specific thing, but rather a collection.

If you end up falling in love with a specific activity, training at the gym may become less of a priority, and playing evolves into training. For example, you might pick up rock climbing and initially only go a few times a month. But after a while you decide to take it more seriously and go more often, until you are rock climbing more than going to the gym. You begin studying the wall to approach it more efficiently. You take time to learn and drill new techniques, and eventually you specify your weight room activities to facilitate climbing. In this case, you've found a hobby you are deeply passionate for and now consider rock climbing something that you train. This is great. Going to the gym might end up being what you do once or twice a week to have fun now. Or perhaps your new climbing friends introduce you to disc golf, and now you do that occasionally.

Whether you train for a sport or workout just to get better, explore all kinds of exercise. Don't discriminate anything based on preconceived notions about it being unsafe or silly. You may surprise yourself with how fun snowboarding is, even though you despise the winter's cold weather. Get out of the gym and try something new.

Chapter 5 – Nutrition

Nutrition is the most important factor to making any physical change in the body. There are so many variables at play with trying to accumulate mass and especially with losing fat. Genetics play a very limited portion, perhaps only up to 20%. Of the remainder, 80% of body composition is based on eating and lifestyle, and 20% is physical activity. Diet constitutes how much your body weighs – exercise molds how that weight is distributed. Diet alone can get you to your desired weight, but working out gets you to your desired shape. There are entire books written on the role of food quality and its effects on metabolism, gene expression, and hormone regulation. While food quality is a major factor within a healthy diet, caloric balance is an easy way to begin thinking about what you eat. It isn't the whole answer, because losing weight is more than just calories in versus calories out. But it is the first step in becoming aware of eating habits and looking at nutrition in a new light to come to a better understanding about how the body uses food for energy.

You cannot out exercise poor eating habits. If you neglect to eat better food, you will likely never achieve your goals, especially if they are fat loss based. Performance athletes can get away with eating unhealthily, because they are not solely focused on how their body looks. Likewise, if you do not eat enough, you will never gain any muscle mass, no matter how hard you train. The first part to understanding food as fuel is to learn that your body takes in energy in the form of kilocalories from food and uses it for all bodily processes. (Calories with a capital "C" is the equivalent to 1000 calories and is the notation you see on food labels. A calorie with a lower case "c" represents 1/1000 of a Calorie or kilocalorie. In reality, a 2000 Calorie diet is the same as a 2,000,000 calorie diet. To be accurate, the term kilocalorie will be used to prevent confusion.) The body uses energy even if you are lying in bed for 24 hours a day, 365 days a year. This is called the basal metabolic rate, or the amount of energy required just to sustain life's physiological processes. All activity, including mental and emotional, adds to the amount of energy you require. In a simple energy balance equation, if you eat more kilocalories than your body uses, you will gain weight. Eating equal kilocalories to kilocalories burned results in no weight gain or loss. And eating less kilocalories than the body requires results in weight loss. (Remember, this is just the first factor in weight regulation.)

You can find free online calculators that provide your basal metabolic rate based on your age, sex, weight, and height. Feel free to use them, however they are only accurate within a degree. The best way to determine how much you should eat is to honestly record everything you eat and count the kilocalories you are consuming for 3-5 days. During these days, just eat as you normally would, because you're looking to find where you may need to make changes in your current habits. There is no point to this project if you lie to yourself and change your patterns to look good on paper. Each morning, weigh yourself. Despite what you may have heard about the negative psychological effects of weighing yourself, due to the body's natural fluctuation on a daily basis, the point in this multiple day experiment is to find a trend in your body's current state. After your 3-5 days eating normally, tracking your kilocalories, and recording your bodyweight, you should conclude a ballpark energy balance. From here, you can now make adjustments accordingly.

If your weight stayed about the same for the past few days, your caloric consumption was also probably pretty steady. If you gained a little weight, you now know you need to eat less kilocalories to come back to a balance. Likewise if you lost weight, you should see that reflected in your food log. If you want to lose weight, start by subtracting 300-500 kilocalories from your benchmark caloric consumption. If you want to gain weight, add 300-500 kilocalories. From here, check in either every day or once a week with your scale to see if you've made progress. The goal is to gradually proceed in the direction of your goals. Fat loss is best sustained at a rate of about 1-2lbs a week[11], or perhaps a little less depending on how much weight you have to lose. If you starve yourself, you will only cause metabolic damage and stall your progress. Muscle however is a much slower game. Physiologically, despite anything you have heard, the male body can only synthesize up to about 1-2lbs of lean muscle in a single month.[12] You might know a guy who claims to have added 5lbs of pure muscle in a month, but it's not physically possible. The weight he has accumulated is partially muscle, water, glycogen, fat, and exaggeration. Elite bodybuilders are elated to have gained 10lbs of muscle in a year, and they are truly doing it with nearly no fat gain either. For women, the rate of muscle synthesis is slower due to lower levels of growth hormone and testosterone.

But what about the notion that if you're working out, you're building muscle while losing fat, so the scale weight isn't going to change? This is true, but only to a small extent. Let's do the math. A 21 year old woman that weights 150lbs at 25% body fat wants to get back to her high school weight of 135lbs. At 150lbs and her current body fat percentage, she is carrying 37.5lbs of fat. With proper resistance training, high intensity cardio, and best case scenario, she loses 0lbs of muscle in her weight loss process. When she reaches her targeted 135lbs after a few months, she has lost 15lbs of hopefully pure fat. This puts her at 16% body fat, or 22.5lbs of fat mass. It is impossible for her weight to remain the same while transitioning from 25% to 16% body fat. In order for her weight to stay at 150lbs while losing fat and gaining muscle, she would have to gain 15lbs of muscle. As stated earlier, that rate of muscle growth is unachievable.

Furthermore, remember when we said it is difficult to accomplish multiple fitness goals at once? The typical new guy at the gym wants to lose fat, gain muscle, and get stronger. These goals all

---

[11] Muth, Natalie. "What Are the Guidelines for Percentage of Body Fat Loss?" ACE Fit. December 2, 2009. Accessed October 2, 2015.
    [12] Thibaudeau, Christian. "The Truth About Bulking." Testosterone Nation. September 26, 2006. Accessed October 3, 2015.

require different training programs, though. You cannot gain any significant muscle while losing weight. Why? Because for the body to grow more muscle, it needs supplies in the form of *surplus* energy. To lose fat, the body must be in a *deficit* of energy. These are counterintuitive physical changes. You may be getting stronger while losing weight, yet this is little to do with gaining muscle, but largely attributed to the nervous system's adaptations associated with strength.

Stepping on the scale isn't the only way to note progress, however. Looking in the mirror reflects the efficacy of your current program. To supplement your markers of change, measuring the circumference of various body parts reveals body composition transformations as well.

Carbohydrates (glucose) get stored in muscles in the form of glycogen. This is a source of energy for muscles during much of physical activity within typical workouts. As you make your muscle contract repeatedly, glycogen gets used up. It is important to note that for each gram of glycogen within a muscle, there are 3 grams of water associated with it.[13] So, when you reduce carbohydrate intake as you try to lose weight (more on this later), three times of the amount of weight lost from glycogen is water. Therefore, as you lose weight, you are losing fat, water, and glycogen (but hopefully not muscle). This is why crash diets have so much "success". What the marketing agents don't tell you is that starving yourself is a great way to deplete glycogen stores, which portrays the illusion of fat loss. Once you begin eating normally, not only are your hormones jacked up from the harsh diet, but you gain back natural levels of glycogen and water.

Reverse this process for those who are packing on muscle. As you gain 1lb of lean mass in an ideal situation, you are also storing more glycogen within that new muscle tissue, and therefore more water.

---

[13] Samuels, Mike. "Glycogen and Weight Loss." LIVESTRONG.COM. May 4, 2014. Accessed October 3, 2015.

This is how someone can claim to gain 5lbs of lean body mass in a month. They aren't just gaining muscle, they are storing more water and glycogen (and probably some fat) too.

Macronutrients

If you paid attention to the nutrition labels while you tracked your kilocalories for the 3-5 days, you should have noticed protein, carbohydrates, and fat values. Food isn't simply comprised of calories. All food contains different amounts of the three macronutrients, protein, carbs, and fat. They serve different purposes in the body and carry varying energy.

Protein

Nearly every physical structure in the body is built by protein. Skin, lungs, stomach, intestines, and of course, muscles, all need adequate protein to maintain normal function and repair. Protein itself is made up of amino acids. There are 20 amino acids available as building blocks to all of the body's structures and functions, 11 of which the body can make. Therefore, 9 amino acids are referred to as essential, meaning the body does not make them and must obtain them from the diet. If a food contains all 9 essential amino acids, it is deemed to be complete. Animal protein sources like meat, fish, and eggs are all complete sources of protein. Vegans must combine foods strategically in order to supply the body with various sources of protein to meet the essential amino acid requirements.

1 gram of protein packs 4 kilocalories (Calories). Though it contains energy, consider protein as the necessary resource for repairing and building biological tissues. The American College of Sports Medicine recommends strength athletes consume 1.6-1.7 grams per kilogram of bodyweight and endurance athletes to eat 1.2-1.4 grams per kilogram of bodyweight.[14] In standard units, that translates to about

0.72 grams and 0.59 grams per pound of bodyweight respectively. Regardless of losing weight or gaining weight, protein is going to be a relatively constant value. You want to maintain the required amounts of protein while in a caloric deficit to retain all possible muscle mass. When training for muscle hypertrophy, excess protein is acceptable, however the body can only absorb a limited quantity, so going far over the recommended amount serves little benefits.

Abundant protein sources are animal meat, eggs, nuts, seeds, and legumes.

Carbohydrates

Carbohydrates are a major source of energy for the body, used in both anaerobic and aerobic exercise. Made of sugars, carbohydrates get broken down into glucose before entering the bloodstream. Insulin is a blood sugar regulating hormone and shuttles glucose into the cells for energy utilization and into the muscles to be stored as glycogen. This process lowers blood sugar levels. Getting insulin and glucose into muscle cells is important for muscle repair and growth. However, once glycogen stores are filled, excess sugar gets stored as fat, which makes walking the razor's edge of managing insulin between too little and too much a path of prudence. An overload of glucose in the bloodstream increases insulin secretion, expedites fat storage, and overall desensitizes cells from responding to the signals of insulin, resulting in type II diabetes.[15]

Carbs also contain 4 kilocalories per gram, but they are digested easier than protein, which gives them more net energy. The thermogenic effect of digestion is the concept that it takes energy to digest food. Proteins take the most energy to digest, while carbs

---

[14] Stoler, Felicia. "ACSM | Sports Nutrition Un-Plugged." ACSM.org. Accessed October 3, 2015.

[15] Hyght, Clay. "The Insulin Advantage." Testosterone Nation. February 14, 2011. Accessed October 3, 2015.

are easier. Plants are mainly carbohydrates. Fruits contain more carbohydrates, hence their sweet taste, and vegetables are mostly carbohydrates in the form of fiber. When eating whole foods, sugar intake is relatively self-moderating. Carbohydrate needs are dependent on goals. Bodybuilders and high level performance athletes with low fat levels can benefit from larger amounts of carbohydrates to facilitate muscle growth and restore the glycogen that is depleted during intense workouts. For these people, consuming 40-60% of calories from carbohydrates (take 40-60% of total calorie allotment and divide by 4 to get amount of carbohydrates in grams) is a good estimate. Those who wish to lose fat should keep carbohydrates lower to allow the body to run through glycogen stores which allows them to tap into fat for energy, as well as keep insulin levels low to prevent more fat accumulation. Staying below 40% of total calories from carbohydrates is a good starting point for this category of trainees, which is very manageable.

Sources of carbohydrates include fruits, grains, nuts, seeds, and vegetables. Of course, processed junk food is primarily refined sugar, which is the most deviant of saccharides.

Fat

Don't let popular media fool you into believing fat makes you fat or causes heart disease. The aforementioned covers that excess sugar is what drives high insulin levels and converts unused carbohydrates into fat. Animal fat (saturated fat) and plant based fats (unsaturated fats) are all very healthy. The only lipid you should avoid that causes serious health problems is trans-fat, a variety that has literally been transformed by hydrogenation to be shelf stable. It is extremely rare in nature, and causes oxidative stress to the body which can lead to numerous illnesses, including heart disease. Recently, the FDA has placed a ban on trans-fats.[16]

---

[16] Sifferlin, Alexandra. "This Is Why FDA Is Banning Trans Fats." Time. June 6, 2105. Accessed October 3, 2015.

Fats are made of a phospholipid head and three fatty acid tails, which is why they are sometimes referred to as phospholipids. They are the most energy dense macronutrient, weighing in at 9 kilocalories per gram. Triglycerides are also the most easily digested nutrient, which makes them extremely efficient for energy utilization. But just because they pack more than double the amount of energy than protein and carbohydrates and are absorbed the easiest, don't shy away from them. During oxidative phosphorylation, a type of aerobic respiration that occurs in a state of depleted glycogen and low intensity movement (walking and regular daily activities) fat is the main source of fuel. Fat is very important for the nervous system, as neurons are coated with fatty sheaths, and cholesterol is the building material for hormones, including testosterone. For those that are trying to lose weight, dietary fat should be a main source of nutrition, and may comprise up to 50% of total calories. The best way to approach how much fat anybody needs is to first meet your protein and carbohydrate requirements and fill the rest of the daily caloric budget with fat. This strategy applies for fat loss, hypertrophy, and strength.

Healthy sources of fat include animal fats, eggs, nuts, seeds, avocados, coconuts, coconut oil, and olive oil. Vegetable oil, canola oil, and some others can be unstable and easily oxidize, causing deleterious health effects. Sticking to animal fats, whole food plant sources, and olive oil or coconut oil leaves you with an abundance of choices. Coconut oil is very stable and therefore great for cooking, because it doesn't break down at high heats. Olive oil is less stable at heat, so it is best used raw, directly on cooked food.

Food Quality

If you take make no dietary changes besides counting calories and macronutrients, you can make good progress, but likely not towards optimum health. IIFYM (if it fits your macros) is a popular nutritional strategy amongst physique athletes because they can achieve desired body compositions with a very flexible diet. Low quality, processed foods are put into any macronutrient parameters, and nutrients such as vitamins and minerals are usually supplemented. This isn't the best way to eat for health. Being fit is more than just body composition or strength – upgrading the organic machine that is your body requires optimal physiological function. The body needs more than just protein, carbs, and fat to survive. These are just fuel sources and basic building blocks. Vitamins and minerals are the micronutrients that are used for chemical processes of all cellular functions. You can supply your cells with all the sugar it needs for energy, but without vitamins and minerals, the cells won't perform properly or at all. Flexible dieting is a great tool at your disposal. It comes in handy when eating out with friends, grabbing something in a pinch, while traveling, or treating yourself. People trying to gain weight can get away with IIFYM much easier because they have more calories with which to work. Eating 4 slices of pizza may only account for 1000 kilocalories in a bodybuilder's 3500 Calorie diet, which means he has plenty of space left for high quality food. A dude looking to lose 15lbs might only be on a 2300 kilocalorie diet, and therefore 1000 kilocalories in pizza might fit very well into his macros, but leaves him little room for high quality food. Most processed foods are very high in kilocalories, so eating a small slice of cake might take a big chunk out of a daily allotment of energy, but doesn't even come close to filling you up. Likewise, a massive salad of kale, spinach, lettuce, peppers, olives, tomatoes, and grilled chicken might only be 500 kilocalories, but fills you up to the brim.

When it comes to getting enough vitamins and minerals, food quality matters. The planet provides everything a biological organism needs for survival. Eating real food is fundamentally all that is required to obtain the nutrients your body requires. The problem is that modern society has turned food into prepackaged, overly processed and refined garbage that is devoid of nutrients. Junk food tastes good because it is loaded with either sugar, salt, or fat. If your diet doesn't consist of lots of vegetables, fruit, and quality meat, then your tastes are probably conditioned to high levels of salt and sugar and may find real, earth grown food to be unappetizing. It's going to take effort and time to retrain your taste buds to appreciate the simple but powerful flavors of natural food.

The best thing you can do to normalize hormones, metabolism, gut bacteria, and energy is to simply eat real food. If doesn't grow or wasn't alive, limit your consumption. Eating more plants increases fiber intake, which in turn will improve blood sugar regulation, digestion and absorption of nutrients. Consuming a variety of colors, or "eating the rainbow" ensures you are feeding yourself a variety of nutrients and covering your bases.

Interesting research about the bacteria that live in the large intestine illuminates the fact that there is more DNA in bacteria in our guts than in our cells collectively. The species and health of the gut microbiome has been shown to drastically effect the physiology of the human body, meaning the bacteria in our intestines actually dictate how our genes are expressed. It might sound crazy, but a certain kind of bacteria called firmicutes was shown to be related to increased fat production. Another kind of bacteria called bacteroides was associated with leanness. In a study with mice given the same amount of calories, those injected with firmicutes bacteria gained fat.[17] This points to the quandary of calories in versus calories out strategy being just a small player in the health game. The good news is that eating a plant based diet naturally facilitates the growth of the lean bacteria, but processed foods support proliferation of the fat-causing bugs.

The final step to having a so-called "clean" diet is to stock up on organic meat and produce. American agricultural practices are highly debated. GMOs, pesticides, fertilizers, and hormones have been nationally sanctioned as safe, but much research contradicts these findings. Most research claims these chemicals have no negative effects on human cells, which is partially true. New

---

[17] Brandt, LJ, and SJ Kallus. "The Intestinal Microbiota and Obesity." National Center for Biotechnology Information. 2012. Accessed October 3, 2015.

findings, however, show that these artificial substances have deleterious effects on the gut bacteria, which we learned plays a major role in how our body functions.[18] This means the chemicals have secondary effects on the body's function, as well as direct consequences. Hormones and antibiotics fed to livestock to force them to quickly grow bigger end up in our bodies. This contributes to medical antibiotics being less affective when we are ill and disrupts our natural hormonal balance (which contributes to weight gain). Without getting too deep into the debate over industrial farming practices, it is fact that grain fed meat has lower levels of omega-3s (an anti-inflammatory essential fatty acid) and higher levels of omega-6s (an inflammatory essential fatty acid). Grass fed meat naturally brings these levels closer to the ideal 1:2 (omega-3 : omega-6) ratio that the body needs for optimal cellular function.[19]

If spending the extra cash on organic food is out of your budget or concerns, at least eating more real foods is a huge step towards feeling and performing your best. If you do want to clean up your diet as best as possible but have trouble with a food budget or accessing all organic options, prioritize organic, grass fed meat. Animal fats store the harmful hormones and antibiotics more than plants store pesticides and fertilizer. Procuring food from local farm markets can be a great way to get more ethically grown food and expose yourself to seasonal produce.

As a final note on food, let's talk about drinks. The only liquid the body needs is water. Staying hydrated is imperative to a well-running machine. You don't need to do any fancy calculations to learn how much water you need – just look in the toilet. If your urine is bright or dark yellow, drink up. You don't need clear urine either, as this might be too much water and result in flushing out the important nutrients you are trying to get with your new, healthy

---

[18] Ji, Sayer. "How GMO Farming and Food Is Making Our Gut Flora UNFRIENDLY." Green Med Info. March 28, 2013. Accessed October 3, 2015.

[19] Ballantyne, Sarah. *The Paleo Approach: Reverse Autoimmune Disease and Heal Your Body*. 86-87.

diet. A light yellow is ideal. Studying your pee will show if you need to drink more or less.

Juice is full of added sugars. Even if it is freshly squeezed from a fruit with no added sugar, separating the naturally occurring sugars from the pulp can be problematic for blood sugar. Imagine how many oranges you would need to eat to get an equivalent amount of an 8oz glass of orange juice. Freshly squeezed juice is fine on occasion, but if you want fruit juice, it's best to just eat the fruit in its whole form.

Alcohol contains 7 kilocalories per gram, which makes it a very dense energy source, except for the fact that the body doesn't get any physiological benefits from alcohol. This is why beer guts exist. Besides having empty calories, the toxic effects of alcohol are widely known. If you enjoy alcohol, consume it moderately.

Nutrition is far more complex than this short chapter, but what is discussed in this book should serve as a crash course in better understanding your body and how to begin feeding it properly. If some of the information seemed surprising, there are many in depth books that speak directly to some of your possible concerns.

Chapter 6 - Rest and Recovery

You can be the hardest worker in the gym, but if you don't give your body an opportunity to rest, recover, and repair, you are digging yourself into the ground. Nutrition plays a big role in getting the body the resources it needs, physically. But, things like rest, sleep, and stress management are just as important to a better body.

The body uses two types of nervous system responses. The sympathetic nervous system is the stress response – it tells the body to run or fight. All stressors trigger this neural response, including exercise, and causes increased heart rate, reaction time, blood flow, and breathing rate by hormonal pathways (largely adrenals such as cortisol, epinephrine, norepinephrine, and adrenaline). Training hard compounded with daily stressors such as lack of sleep, problems at work or at home, and general irritants all activate the sympathetic nervous system and tell the body to prepare for battle.

On the other hand, the parasympathetic is the rest and digest nervous system response. It's associated with slow, deep breathing, reduced heart rate, being calm, sleeping, and digesting. This is the state the body needs to be in to recover and repair from the stressors that stimulate the sympathetic nervous system. The problem is, life is full of stressful situations, and exercise only adds to it. In order to enhance your body, you are going to have to take a few steps to activate the parasympathetic nervous system and chill out.

First of all, you don't have to train every single day to reach your goals. There are daily training regimens that are quite demanding, but they are reserved for elite athletes that are already in great condition and whose bodies are adapted to this stimulus. For the general public, especially those of you who are new to exercise, training 3-5 days a week is plenty. Giving your body a few days each week to cool out and recover is important. This is the time where damaged tissue can repair microtrauma and make all the favorable adaptations you seek. Not only are physical changes made on rest days, but the central nervous system can quiet down after bouts of heavy lifting and neural demand.

Getting enough sleep is paramount to recovery and stress management. The body and brain go through all kinds of healing and reset during sleep. Getting 7.5-9 hours of sleep is ideal. Because brain activity occurs in 90 minute cycles during sleep, waking up within a 90 minute cycle can result in feeling groggy in the morning. By sleeping through the full 90 minute period, the body wakes up feeling refreshed, instead of interrupted. This is why sleeping 7.5 hours can feel better than 8.[20]

Besides getting a good night's rest, doing anything you can to relax will facilitate recovery and a reduction in the stress response.

Revisiting mobility with static stretching and soft tissue work such as foam rolling or going to a masseuse for a deep tissue massage will help with recovery. Not only will these activities relax your mind and body, but help with performance. Pumping metabolic waste out of the muscles, increasing blood flow, working out knots, and decreasing neural tone are advantageous.

---

[20] "Natural Patterns of Sleep." Healthysleep.med.harvard.edu. December 18, 2007. Accessed October 6, 2015.

Conclusions

Choosing quality movement is the best way to address physical fitness. Resistance training via the basic human movement patterns is so adaptable, which makes it the ideal modality for fat loss, muscle growth, strength, and cardio. Manipulating training variables in accordance to your specificities is what makes programming unique to every person. You might need to do high reps with very short rest, or few reps with long rest. But by moving your body based on its anatomical design, you will learn to move better, feel better, and live better. Scale makes all movement patterns accessible, regardless of skill level. Choose an exercise for each variation based on your current aptitude, and challenge yourself to move towards difficult progressions over time.

Physical training isn't all about hard work. Get outside and express your new body in fun ways that aren't available in a weight room. Finding a group of friends with whom you can work out and enjoy a host of other physical activities makes adherence stronger. When you enjoy something you are more apt to stick with it. You may begin viewing your time in the gym as preparation for your new hobby. Have fun and move your body whenever an opportunity is presented.

Dietary and lifestyle habits are a major chunk of the game. You can't outrun a fork, and you only add to stress with physical exertion. Adopting healthy nutritional habits by eating real food is the best thing you can do to begin nourishing your meat robot for optimal performance. Getting enough rest and not worrying about trivialities clears the mind to better handle more important problems, instead of revving up over a collection of minor issues.

Begin shifting your perspective to that which sees the human body as an organic machine. The body's anatomy is like the suspension, wheels, brakes, nuts, and bolts of a car. The nervous system and physiology is the driver behind the wheel. In order to win the race, you naturally will install the best modifications for your car and hire the most skilled driver with the best reaction time. Treat your body right and stack the cards in your favor.

Sample Programs

Bodyweight Basics:

Three days a week, every other day (ie. Monday, Wednesday, Friday), perform the following three exercises for 5 sets.

- Pull Ups (or Inverted Row)
- Pushups (or incline progression)
- Squat/Lunge

Just like the pushup progression mentioned in Chapter 3, do X amount of reps for 5 sets. For example, do 5 sets of 1 rep for pull up. The next workout, attempt 5 sets of 2 reps. If you fall short with a scheme of 2,2,1,1,1, continue adding reps to your last three sets, until you achieve 5x2. Continue with 3 reps for 5 sets and so forth. Use this strategy to build strength with all your bodyweight movements. For the lower body exercises, you will likely approach upwards of 20 repetitions. This is fine, as you will be developing your cardiovascular system while building a solid base of strength and muscle mass in your legs. You can always choose harder lower body variations with pistol squats or broad jumps. Depending on your rep range, take varying rest intervals. For pull ups, you will likely need 2+ minutes between sets. If you can do 8 or more reps, choose 60-90 second rest periods. If you get more than 15 reps, rest no more than 30-60 sets.

This is a great program for all beginners to start, because there is little investment required and you will learn how to control your own body. Make a one-time purchase of a doorframe pull up bar for about $20 (add in a pair of gymnastics rings for $30 for inverted rows), and you've got a home gym. This is a quick way to fit an incredibly affective workout into a busy schedule.

3 Day Alternating Full Body Hypertrophy

Once you've mastered your own body, you can move on to lifting weights. At this point, you should have a solid base of strength and muscle, along with a new passion for physical activity. Still being three days of lifting, this program leaves plenty of time for additional cardio, play time, or whatever else you want to do. Great for building muscle mass and establishing form with lifting external loads, implement this three day program by alternating the two workouts every other day. For instance, the first week will be workout A, B, A. The next week will follow as workout B, A, B. It repeats like this continuously, three days a week, every other day. Choose a weight that allows you to complete the 5x10 scheme, with a 60-120 second rest interval. Progress just like the bodyweight routine. Don't move up in weight until you reach the 5 sets of 10. Every fourth or fifth week, consider taking a deload. Either take the entire week to rest, do light cardio, or just less sets or weight. This gives your body an extended period to recovery and prevent overtraining.

Workout A:
- Squat (5x10)
- Overhead Press (5x10)
- Pull Up (5 sets of X)

Workout B:
- Deadlift (5x10)
- Bench Press (5x10)
- Barbell Row (5x10)

4 Day Lower/Upper Body Hypertrophy

This workout plan is 2 days on, 2 days off (ie. Mon, Tues, Thurs, Fri). By splitting the lower and upper body into two training sessions each, you can work each muscle group harder and have more potential for hypertrophy.

Lower Body 1:
- Squat (5x10)
- Deadlift (5x10)
- Lunge (5x10)

Upper Body 1:
- Bench Press (5x10)
- Pull Up (5 sets of X)
- Pushups (5 sets of X)
- Barbell Row (5x10)

Lower Body 2:
- Deadlift (5x10)
- Squat (5x10)
- Step Ups (5x10)

Upper Body 2:
- Overhead Press (5x10)
- Pull Up (5 sets of X)
- Incline Bench Press (5x10)
- Dumbbell Row (5x10)

3 Day Alternating Full Body 5x5 Strength

Similar to the 3 day hypertrophy split, this takes the same core movements but uses strength parameters. Due to the lifts being heavier, use a 2-3 minute rest interval.

Workout A:
- Squat (5x5)
- Bench Press (5x5)
- Pull Up (5x5) Add weight if needed with a weight belt.

Workout B:
- Deadlift (5x5)
- Overhead Press (5x5)
- Barbell Row (5x5)

Bibliography

Ballantyne, Sarah. *The Paleo Approach: Reverse Autoimmune Disease and Heal Your Body.* 86-87.

Brandt, LJ, and SJ Kallus. "The Intestinal Microbiota and Obesity." National Center for Biotechnology Information. 2012. Accessed October 3, 2015.

"Butt Wink Is Not About the Hamstrings - DeanSomerset.com." DeanSomersetcom. July 7, 2014. Accessed September 30, 2015.

Contreas, Bret. "The Hypertrophy Specialist." Testosterone Nation. October 27, 2010. Accessed September 29, 2015. https://www.t-nation.com/training/hypertrophy-specialist.

Cressey, Eric, and Mike Robertson. "Feel Better for 10 Bucks." Testosterone Nation. July 12, 2004. Accessed September 29, 2015. https://www.t-nation.com/training/feel-better-for-10-bucks.

Dumitru, Luminița, Alina Iliescu, Cristian Dumitru, Ruxandra Badea, Simona Săvulescu, Horațiu Dinu, and Mihai Berteanu. 2014. "Physiological considerations on Neuromuscular Electrical Stimulation (NMES) in muscular strength training." Palestrica Of The Third Millennium Civilization & Sport 15, no. 2: 134-139. Academic Search Complete, EBSCOhost (accessed September 29, 2015).

Gentilcore, Tony. "Soft Tissue Work for Tough Guys." Testosterone Nation. September 19, 2006. Accessed September 29, 2015. https://www.t-nation.com/training/soft-tissue-work-for-tough-guys.

Hyght, Clay. "The Insulin Advantage." Testosterone Nation. February 14, 2011. Accessed October 3, 2015.

Ji, Sayer. "How GMO Farming and Food Is Making Our Gut Flora UNFRIENDLY." Green Med Info. March 28, 2013. Accessed October 3, 2015.

Muth, Natalie. "What Are the Guidelines for Percentage of Body Fat Loss?" ACE Fit. December 2, 2009. Accessed October 2, 2015.

"Natural Patterns of Sleep." Healthysleep.med.harvard.edu. December 18, 2007. Accessed October 6, 2015.

Ogden CL, Carroll MD, Kit BK, Flegal KM. Prevalence of Childhood and Adult Obesity in the United States, 2011-2012. *JAMA*.2014;311(8):806-814. doi:10.1001/jama.2014.732.

Samuels, Mike. "Glycogen and Weight Loss." LIVESTRONG.COM. May 4, 2014. Accessed October 3, 2015.

Shugart, Chris. "Predator Conditioning." Testosterone Nation. October 28, 2013. Accessed September 28, 2015. https://www.t-nation.com/training/predator-conditioning.

Sifferlin, Alexandra. "This Is Why FDA Is Banning Trans Fats." Time. June 6, 2105. Accessed October 3, 2015.

Stoler, Felicia. "ACSM | Sports Nutrition Un-Plugged." ACSM.org. Accessed October 3, 2015.

"Stress Effects on The Body." Apa.org. Accessed September 29, 2015. http://www.apa.org/helpcenter/stress-body.aspx.

Thibaudeau, Christian. "The Truth About Bulking." Testosterone
    Nation. September 26, 2006. Accessed October 3, 2015.

Tumminello, Nick. "A Simple Program for Complex Results."
    Testosterone Nation. December 10, 2010. Accessed October
    3, 2015.